Chapter 1 : Nutritional imbalance

Importance of a balanced diet

Balanced diet is crucial for overall health. It relies on variety and balance, providing all the essential nutrients for the body. Key nutrients include proteins for tissue repair, carbohydrates for energy, lipids for cell health, as well as vitamins and minerals for the body's proper functioning. A balanced diet helps maintain a healthy weight, strengthens the immune system, and reduces the risks of chronic diseases such as heart disease and diabetes.

Example of a Balanced Daily Meal Plan:

Breakfast: Oatmeal with fresh fruit and nuts.
Lunch: Quinoa salad with various vegetables and grilled chicken.
Snack: Natural yogurt with berries.
Dinner: Salmon fillet, steamed vegetables, and sweet potato.

Meal Planning

Planning your meals is essential for maintaining a balanced diet. Start by identifying your personal nutritional needs. Use tools like the USDA's MyPlate to understand the ideal proportions of each food group on your plate.
Plan your meals by including a variety of foods: fruits, vegetables, proteins, whole grains, and dairy products. Preparing meals in advance can prevent impulsive choices and promote a healthy and balanced diet.

Meal Planning Tips:

Prepare a shopping list based on your weekly meal plan.
Consider batch cooking on the weekend to save time.
Vary your protein sources among meat, fish, legumes, and tofu.

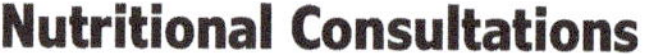

Nutritional Consultations

Nutritionists are essential for establishing a personalized and balanced diet. They assess your nutritional needs, eating habits, and lifestyle to develop a tailored plan. Consultations also help manage specific conditions like gluten intolerance or diabetes. They provide ongoing support and diet adjustments based on your progress and life changes.

Benefits of Nutritional Consultations:

Identification of nutritional deficiencies.
Personalized advice based on your health and goals.
Continuous support and motivation.

Nutritional Tracking

Using nutritional tracking apps can be a powerful tool. These apps help you monitor your daily nutrient and calorie intake, providing an overview of your eating habits. They can also offer meal suggestions and healthy recipes.

Recommended Apps:

MyFitnessPal: For tracking calories and physical activities.
Cronometer: For detailed nutrient analysis.
Yazio: For meal planning and health goal tracking.

Case Studies and Testimonials

Including testimonials from women who have improved their health through nutritional balance can be very inspiring. These personal stories provide insight into challenges and successes, making the path to better health more relatable and accessible.

Example of Testimony:

<u>Testimony 1:</u> Dietary Course Change
"Laura, 42, an architect, long struggled with balancing her diet. She often ate on the go and favored fast, low-nutrient foods. After realizing the impact of her diet on her health and well-being, she began to plan her meals and include more fruits and vegetables. 'It was a gradual change, but the effects were immediate,' she explains. 'I feel more energetic, my skin is healthier, and I've even improved my concentration at work.'"

<u>Testimony 2:</u> Breakfast Revolution
"Sophie, 35, a nurse and mother of two, long neglected breakfast, settling for a quick coffee. After learning the importance of a balanced breakfast, she started integrating protein smoothies and avocado toast into her morning routine. 'It was a revelation,' she says. 'I have more energy all day, and I snack less. My mood has improved, and I feel stronger to handle my busy days.'"

<u>Testimony 3:</u> Discovering the Joys of Cooking
"Marie, 48, a marketing director, always resorted to prepared meals due to lack of time. When she began experiencing health problems related to her unbalanced diet, she decided to enroll in a cooking class. 'Learning to cook changed my life,' she shares. 'I now enjoy preparing healthy meals. Not only has my health improved, but these moments in the kitchen have become my new form of meditation.'"

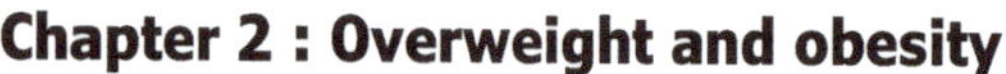

Chapter 2 : Overweight and obesity

Understanding overweight and obesity

Overweight and obesity are defined by an excess of body fat that can be detrimental to health. These conditions often result from an energy imbalance between calories consumed and calories expended. Factors include genetics, metabolism, environment, lifestyle, and eating habits. Associated risks include type 2 diabetes, heart diseases, certain cancers, and joint problems.

Key Statistics (CDC, 2023):

About 35% of American women aged 20 and older are obese.
The obesity rate increases with age, reaching 40% among those aged 40-59.

Exercise and Physical Activity

Physical activity is essential for
weight control and overall health improvement. Regular exercise helps burn excess calories, strengthens the heart and muscles, and improves mood and energy.

Adapted Exercise Programs:

For beginners: Brisk walking, swimming, yoga.
For intermediate level: Jogging, cycling, group fitness classes.
For advanced: High-Intensity Interval Training (HIIT), weight training.

Diet and Portion Control

A healthy diet for weight management includes a variety of foods in appropriate quantities. Eating diverse fruits, vegetables, whole grains, lean proteins, and limiting high-fat and sugary foods is essential.

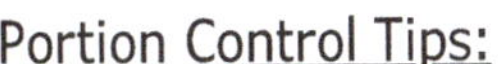

<u>Portion Control Tips:</u>

Use smaller plates to reduce portion sizes.
Do not eat directly from the package, but serve a defined portion.
Listen to your body's hunger and satiety signals.

Psychological Support

Emotional support is crucial in the fight against overweight. Therapy, support groups, or wellness coaching can help understand and manage emotional eating habits.

<u>Benefits of Psychological Support:</u>

Improved relationship with food.
Stress and anxiety management related to eating.
Enhanced motivation and self-esteem.

Resources and References

Books: "The Obesity Code" by Dr. Jason Fung, "Mindful Eating" by Jan Chozen Bays.
Websites: Nutrition.gov, ChooseMyPlate.gov.
Apps: Lose It!, Noom.

Testimonials

<u>Testimonial 1:</u> Julia's Journey
"Julia, 37, a teacher, struggled with obesity for years. After incorporating daily walking sessions and adjusting her food portions, she began to see changes. 'I lost 20 kilograms in a year, but more importantly, I gained confidence and vitality,' she shares."

<u>Testimonial 2:</u> Mark's Transformation
"Mark, 45, an engineer, realized the importance of mental health in weight management. By combining a healthy diet with behavioral therapy, he overcame his compulsive eating habits. 'It not only helped me lose weight but also regain mental balance,' he says."

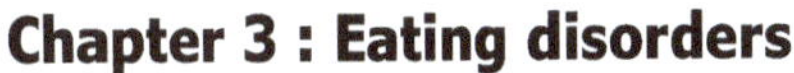

Chapter 3 : Eating disorders

Types and symptoms

Eating disorders, such as anorexia, bulimia, and binge eating disorder, are serious conditions that affect both mental and physical health. Characterized by an obsession with food, weight, and body shape, these disorders can manifest as extreme dietary restrictions, episodes of overeating followed by compensatory behaviors, and uncontrolled food consumption.

Cognitive Behavioral Therapy (CBT)

CBT is a proven method for treating eating disorders. It helps change negative thoughts and behaviors related to eating, body image, and self-esteem by developing emotional management strategies and healthy eating habits.

Support Groups and Group Therapy

Support groups and group therapy provide a safe space to share experiences and resilience strategies. They offer a sense of community and mutual understanding, crucial in the healing process.

Supervised Nutritional Strategies

Collaborating with a nutritionist or dietitian is essential to establish a healthy and balanced diet. These professionals design personalized meal plans that support recovery while ensuring adequate nutrition.

Studies and Resources

Organizations like the National Eating Disorders Association (NEDA) offer information, support, and guidance for those affected by these disorders.

Testimonials

<u>Testimonial 1:</u> Sara's Journey
 "Sara, 28, a teacher, battled bulimia for years. Thanks to a combination of CBT and nutritional support, she was able to redefine her relationship with food. 'It was a difficult journey, but I learned the importance of nourishing my body and mind,' she says."

<u>Testimonial 2:</u> Emma's Renaissance
"Emma, 34, an architect, suffered from anorexia in her youth. By joining a support group and working closely with a nutritionist, she gradually found her way to a healthy diet. 'The support of the community and professional advice were vital in my recovery,' she shares."

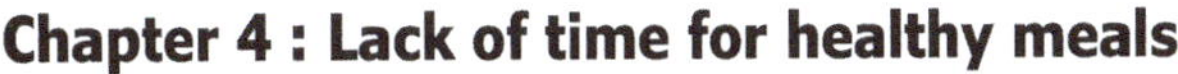

Chapter 4 : Lack of time for healthy meals

Daily challenges

In the bustling life of modern women, balancing career, family, and personal time can make it difficult to prepare healthy meals. Often, the convenience of quick and less nutritious options seems to be the only solution in a tight schedule.

Planning and preparing meals in advance are key to healthy eating despite a busy agenda. Dedicating time during the weekend to prepare dishes can be greatly helpful.

Examples of Balanced Meals to Prepare in Advance:

Roasted Chicken with Quinoa and Broccoli: A combination of lean protein, whole grains, and green vegetables.

Lentil Salad with Spinach and Feta: A meal rich in fiber, iron, and protein.

Burrito Bowls with Brown Rice, Black Beans, and Vegetables: A balanced meal with a good portion of legumes and fresh vegetables.

Vegetable Curry with Tofu: A vegetarian option rich in protein and a variety of vegetables.

Salmon en Papillote with Asparagus and Sweet Potatoes: A complete meal with omega-3s, complex carbohydrates, and vegetables.

Healthy Meal Delivery Services

For those who lack time, healthy meal delivery services offer a convenient alternative, with varied and customizable options to meet specific nutritional needs.

Quick and Nutritious Recipes

Incorporating easy and quick recipes to prepare in less than 30 minutes is crucial for a healthy diet.

Examples of Quick Recipes:

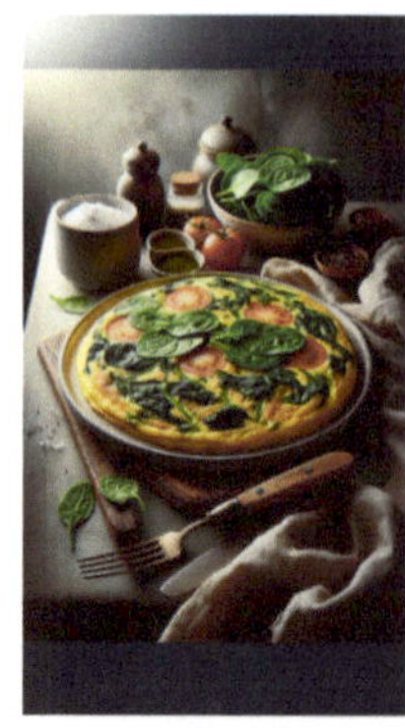

Spinach and Tomato Omelette: High in protein and easy to make for a nourishing breakfast

Chicken and avocado wrap : A quick lunch with a good balance of protein, healthy fats, and vegetables.

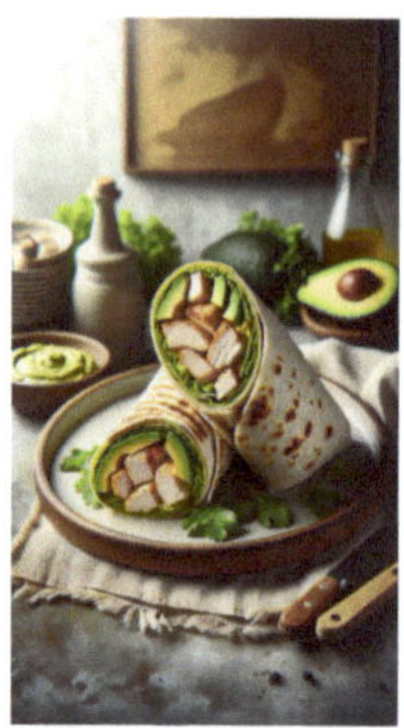

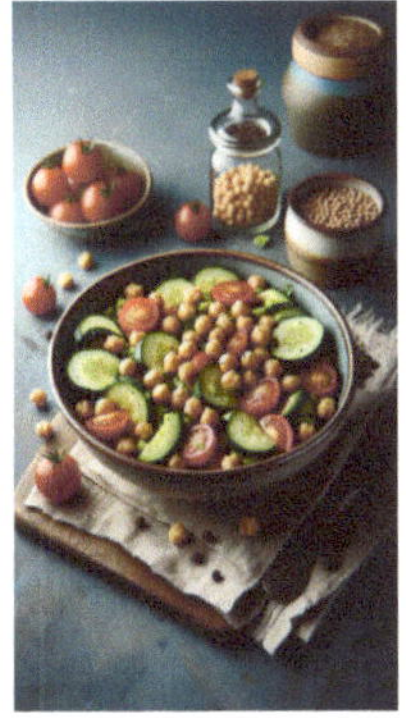

Mediterranean chickpea salad : Ideal for a light lunch or dinner, rich in fiber and protein.

Kale and walnut pesto pasta : A quick dinner, rich in nutrients and flavors.

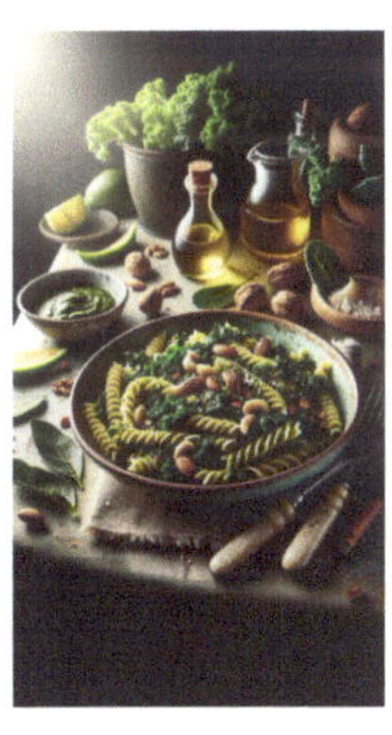

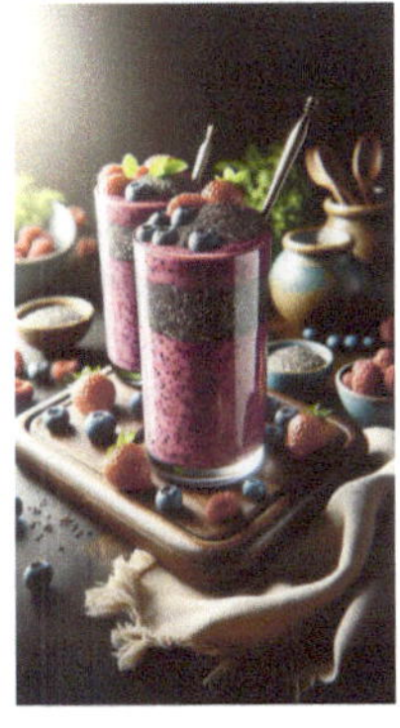

Berry and Chia seed smoothie : Perfect for a quick breakfast or a snack rich in antioxidants and omega-3s.

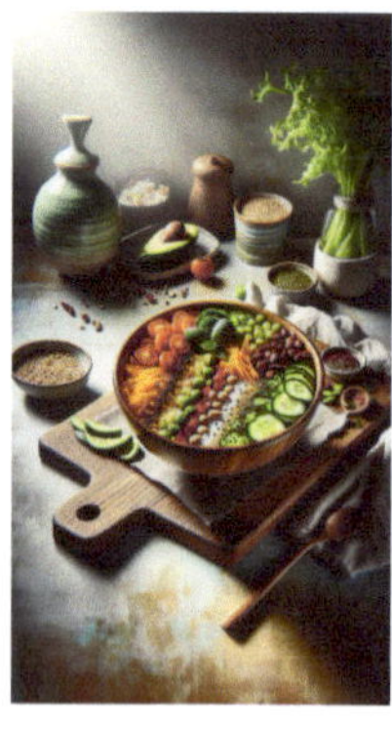

Bouddha bowl: Base of brown rice or quinoa, topped with roasted vegetables (carrots, cauliflower), chickpeas, and drizzled with tahini sauce

Testimonials and Studies

Sharing stories of women who have successfully incorporated healthy meal preparation into their busy routines can motivate and inspire.

Testimonial 1: Laura's Transformation
"Laura, 39, a lawyer, struggled to eat healthily with her busy schedule. By adopting meal prep on Sundays, she changed her eating habits. 'It helped me save time and control my diet.'"

Testimonial 2: Anna's Life Change
"Anna, 36, a marketing consultant, used to skip meals or eat on the go. By starting meal prep, she not only saved time but also improved her diet. 'It completely changed the way I eat. I feel more energetic and healthier,' she shares."

Testimonial 3: Lea's Culinary Revelation
"Lea, 29, a software engineer, found it difficult to eat healthily with a demanding work schedule. Discovering quick and nutritious recipes was a revelation. 'It allowed me to eat better without spending hours in the kitchen,' she says."

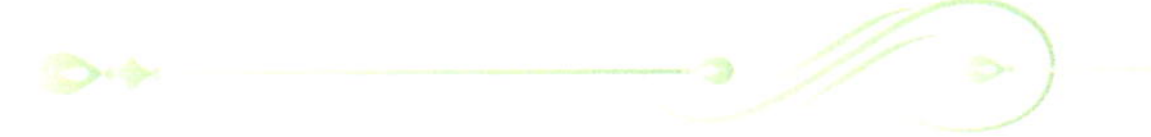

Chapter 5 : Food sensitivities and allergies

Identifying allergies

Food sensitivities and allergies can play a major role in overall well-being. Identifying these allergies is the first step. Symptoms such as bloating, skin rashes, headaches, or digestive issues after eating certain foods may indicate a sensitivity or allergy.

Adapting the Diet

After identifying allergens, it is crucial to adapt the diet to avoid them. This may involve carefully reading food product labels, learning to cook with alternatives, and remaining vigilant during meals outside.

Examples of Dietary Adaptations:

For gluten allergy, opt for gluten-free cereals like quinoa or brown rice. For lactose intolerance, use plant-based milks like almond or soy milk. For nut allergies, substitute with seeds like sunflower or pumpkin seeds.

Reading Labels and Prevention

Knowing how to read labels is essential to avoid allergens.This includes recognizing alternative names for allergens and understanding possible traces of allergens in food products.

Food Alternatives

Exploring food alternatives can open up a new culinary world. For example, for those who cannot consume dairy products, there are a variety of plant-based cheeses and yogurts.

References and Resources

Resources like Food Allergy Research & Education (FARE) or the American College of Allergy, Asthma, and Immunology can provide valuable information and advice for managing food allergies.

Testimonials

<u>Testimonial 1:</u> Isabelle's Discovery
"Isabelle, 41, a graphic designer, suffered from chronic headaches and fatigue. After being diagnosed with gluten sensitivity, she adapted her diet, which greatly improved her quality of life. 'It required adjustments, but I feel so much better now,' she says."

<u>Testimonial 2:</u> Sophie's Journey
"Sophie, 35, a teacher, discovered a nut allergy later in life.

Learning to read labels and discovering safe alternatives allowed her to safely navigate her diet. 'At first, it was intimidating, but now it's become second nature,' she shares."

Chapter 6 : Impact of aging on nutrition and well-being

Nutritional changes with age

As women age, their nutritional needs change. Factors such as a decrease in metabolism, hormonal changes, and a reduction in muscle mass affect caloric and nutritional needs. It becomes important to focus on nutrient-rich foods, such as fruits, vegetables, lean proteins, whole grains, and low-fat dairy products.

Weight Management at Different Ages

Weight control can become more challenging with age due to slowed metabolism and muscle mass loss. Adopting a balanced diet and maintaining regular physical activity are essential for effective weight management.

Importance of Nutrient Density

With age, eating nutrient-dense foods is crucial. This means choosing foods that provide maximum nutrients for a minimum number of calories. For example, leafy green vegetables, fruits, nuts, and whole grains are excellent choices.

Prevention of Age-Related Diseases

A healthy diet plays a key role in preventing age-related diseases such as osteoporosis, heart disease, and type 2 diabetes. Adequate intake of calcium, vitamin D, and fiber are particularly important.

Testimonials and Practical Advice

Sharing testimonials from women who have adapted their diet and lifestyle to meet the challenges of aging can be inspiring and informative.

Testimonial 1: Marie's Adaptation
"Marie, 52, an accountant, noticed her metabolism slowing down with age. By focusing on a diet rich in vegetables, fruits, and whole grains, and practicing brisk walking, she successfully maintained a healthy weight and feels more energetic than ever. 'It's all about adapting and listening to your body,' she explains."

Testimonial 2: Linda's Transformation
"Linda, 60, a retiree, faced health challenges related to menopause. By incorporating more calcium and vitamin D into her diet to strengthen her bones, and staying active, she improved her overall health. 'It's never too late to start taking care of yourself,' she says."

These stories offer unique perspectives on how diet and physical activity can be adjusted to meet the changing needs of women as they age, highlighting the importance of a proactive approach to health and well-being.

Chapter 7 : Managing stress en mental health

Link between diet and mental health

Diet plays a crucial role in mental health. Certain foods can influence mood, energy, and cognition. Diets rich in fruits, vegetables, whole grains, and omega-3 fatty acids are associated with a reduced risk of depression and anxiety.

Diet for Stress Reduction

Specific dietary choices can help manage stress. For example, foods high in magnesium (such as spinach and almonds) and foods rich in vitamin B (such as avocados and whole grains) can help reduce stress levels.

Impact of Eating Habits on Mood

Regular and balanced eating habits support stable mood. Avoiding long periods without eating and excessive sugar can help maintain consistent energy levels and prevent mood swings.

Mindful Eating for Improved Mental Health

Mindful eating, or eating with attention and without distraction, appreciating each bite, and listening to the body's hunger and satiety signals, can improve the relationship with food and help avoid overeating.

Testimonials and Practical Strategies

Incorporating stories of women who have used diet and mindfulness to improve their mental well-being can be very encouraging for readers.

Testimonials

Testimonial 1: Élise Finds Balance
"Élise, 44, an entrepreneur, struggled with stress and anxiety for a long time. By adopting a nutrient-rich diet and practicing mindful eating, she noticed a significant improvement in her mood and stress management. 'It changed the way I see food and life,' she says."

Testimonial 2: Julie's Path to Serenity
"Julie, 38, a nurse, found that regular meals and the choice of healthy foods had a positive impact on her daily mood. By avoiding sugar spikes and crashes, she gained energy and emotional stability. 'It really helped balance my days,' she shares."

These stories highlight how a balanced diet and a mindful approach to eating can play a beneficial role in managing stress and improving mental health.

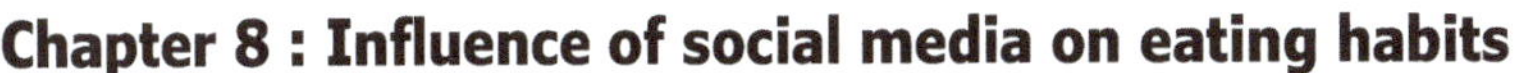

Chapter 8 : Influence of social media on eating habits

Impact of social media on perception of food

Social media can significantly impact how women perceive diet and health. Food trends, beauty ideals, and fashionable diets often promoted on these platforms can create unrealistic expectations and pressure to follow potentially unhealthy eating habits.

Resisting Harmful Food Trends

It is crucial to develop a critical mindset towards food trends promoted on social media. This involves seeking reliable and scientifically based information and being wary of fad diets that promise quick results but are not sustainable or balanced.

Promoting Healthy Eating on Digital Platforms

Using social media positively by following accounts that promote healthy eating, balanced lifestyle habits, and a positive body image can be beneficial. This can help create an inspiring and supportive online environment.

Creating a Support Community

Social media offers the opportunity to join communities sharing similar interests in nutrition and well-being. These communities can provide support, motivation, and share positive experiences.

Testimonials and Practical Advice

Sharing experiences of women who have overcome the negative influence of social media and found balance in their relationship with food can be extremely inspiring.

Testimonials

Testimonial 1: Amélie's Turnaround
"Amélie, 31, a life coach, was influenced by unrealistic diets and images on social media. By becoming aware of their negative impact, she sought reliable information sources and started following realistic nutritionists and life coaches. 'It transformed my perception of health and beauty,' she explains."

Testimonial 2: Caroline's Digital Awakening
"Caroline, 29, a graphic designer, found an online community supporting nutrition and well-being after struggling with body image. Sharing experiences and practical advice helped her adopt a healthier approach to eating. 'It allowed me to free myself from the pressure of social media,' she says."

These testimonials highlight the importance of navigating social media with caution and intention, choosing influences that promote a healthy and balanced approach to diet and well-being.

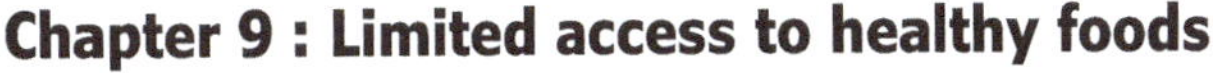

Chapter 9 : Limited access to healthy foods

Disparity in food access

Access to healthy foods varies significantly based on socioeconomic, geographic, and cultural conditions. In some areas, known as food deserts, access to fresh and affordable foods is limited, negatively impacting health and well-being.

Strategies to Overcome Obstacles

For those living in areas where access to healthy foods is limited, there are strategies to incorporate quality nutrition. This can include participating in food cooperatives, cultivating home gardens, or purchasing from local markets.

Utilizing Community Resources

Community resources such as food banks, farmers' markets, and food assistance programs can help bridge the gap in access to healthy food. Participating in these initiatives can also strengthen the social and community fabric.

Nutritional Education

Nutritional education plays a key role in understanding and effectively using available resources. Educational programs can teach how to prepare healthy meals with limited resources.

Testimonials and Case Studies

Stories of women who have overcome challenges in accessing healthy foods can serve as inspiration and provide practical strategies for others in similar situations.

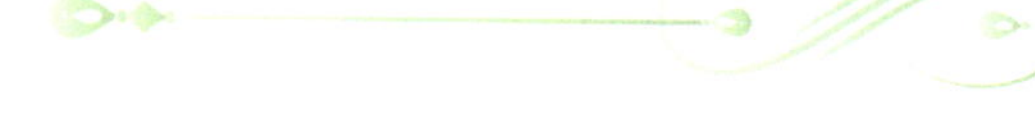

Testimonials

<u>Testimonial 1:</u> Nadia's Initiative
"Nadia, 40, a social worker, lives in an area with limited access to fresh foods. By participating in a community garden and using resources from local farmers' markets, she was able to introduce more fresh fruits and vegetables into her diet. 'It required creativity, but it's very rewarding,' she says."

<u>Testimonial 2:</u> Fatima's Resilience
"Fatima, 35, a stay-at-home mother, had to learn how to feed her family on a tight budget. Thanks to nutritional education programs, she developed skills to prepare healthy and economical meals. 'It helped me better nourish my family despite our limitations,' she shares."

These stories highlight the importance of innovation, using community resources, and education in overcoming obstacles to access healthy foods, particularly in disadvantaged areas.
Haut du formulaire

Chapter 10 : Hormonal change and nutrition

Hormonal impact on metabolism and appetite

Hormonal changes, especially during periods such as pregnancy, menopause, or the menstrual cycle, can significantly affect metabolism, appetite, and fat storage. Understanding these changes is essential to adapt the diet and maintain nutritional balance.

Nutrition Adapted to Different Life Phases

At each stage of a woman's life, her nutritional needs evolve. For example, during pregnancy, the focus is on folic acid, iron, and calcium. During menopause, it is important to support bone health with increased intake of calcium and vitamin D.

Managing Symptoms through Diet

Certain foods can help manage symptoms associated with hormonal changes. For instance, foods rich in phytoestrogens, like soy, can help alleviate menopause symptoms. Foods high in magnesium and vitamin B6 can help reduce premenstrual syndrome (PMS) symptoms.

Importance of Hydration and Exercise

Besides diet, hydration and physical exercise play a crucial role in managing hormonal changes.
Drinking enough water and maintaining regular physical activity can help alleviate certain symptoms and support overall well-being.

Testimonials and Practical Advice

Sharing experiences of women who have adapted their diet in response to hormonal changes can provide valuable advice and a sense of solidarity.

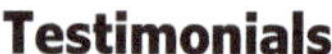

Testimonials

<u>Testimonial 1:</u> Véronique Finds Balance
"Véronique, 51, a teacher, experienced notable changes in her body and mood during menopause. By incorporating more green vegetables and calcium sources into her diet, and increasing her physical activity, she effectively managed her symptoms. 'It made a big difference in my daily life,' she shares."

<u>Testimonial 2:</u> Laura's Transition "Laura, 29, an architect, suffered from severe PMS for years. By changing her diet to include more foods rich in magnesium and B6, she noticed a significant improvement. 'It changed the way I live through these periods,' she says."

These testimonials highlight the importance of understanding and responding to changing nutritional needs related to hormonal fluctuations, offering concrete strategies to maintain balance and well-being.

Conclusion

In this book, "Women's Health," we have explored a wide range of crucial topics for women's health and well-being, from nutritional balance to managing hormonal changes. Through each chapter, we have sought to provide reliable information, practical advice, and inspiring testimonials to help each reader navigate her unique health journey.

Diet and well-being are not just about food choices or physical activity; they are intrinsically linked to our mental health, our social and economic environment, and our physiological changes throughout life. This book aims to equip you not only with knowledge but also with the confidence to make informed and personal health choices.

We hope the strategies and stories shared here will resonate with you and encourage you on your own journey of well-being. Whether you are facing challenges related to diet, stress management, or adapting to hormonal changes, remember that you are not alone. There is immense strength in knowledge and community, and this book aims to be a source of support and inspiration.

Ultimately, "Women's Health" is more than a guide; it's a celebration of resilience, diversity, and the ability of women to thrive through the different phases of their lives. We encourage you to continue learning, experimenting, and finding what works best for you, for your body and your mind. Health is a personal and evolving journey, and we are honored to accompany you at every step of the way.

Take care of yourself, and remember: your health is your greatest wealth.